Yoga for Beginners

A Beginners Guide To Yoga

Disclaimer

All the material contained in this book is
provided for educational and informational
purposes only. No responsibility can be taken
for any results or outcomes resulting from the
use of this material.

While every attempt has been made to provide
information that is both accurate and effective,
the author does not assume any responsibility
for the accuracy or use/misuse of this
information.

Introduction

This book is your entrance to the world of yoga and meditation. Before setting off on this journey, you need to know what yoga is, its history and the philosophy behind it.

Yoga is a physical, spiritual and mental discipline which origins go back to India and to its three famous philosophical beliefs; Hinduism, Buddhism and Jainism.

Yoga in Vedic Sanskrit comes from the root "yuj" means "to add", "to join", "to unite", or "to attach". Most people go for that yoga means "unity" and "connection", and that this unity is meant to be achieved between the body, soul and mind.

1. History

Yoga first appeared in India in the per-Vedic era, by that time it was a broad term that included many schools and philosophies. It discussed morals and how to deal with people, personal observance and the aspects that form our behaviors, unity with the spiritual world and the supreme and finally the physical exercises and positions.

Through the years, the aim of yoga to understand the world started to change and the focus later targeted instead self-enlightenment as the ultimate goal of yoga.

However, when yoga was introduced to the west in 1890s it was mainly concerned with the physical approach and it took people long years to start considering the spiritual part known as meditation.

2. Philosophy

Yoga has many philosophical schools in Hinduism, Buddhism and Jainism. Instead of getting lost in the Vedic Sanskrit names and the principles of each discipline, we will highlight the common general philosophical concepts yoga addresses.

- Unity between the matter and the mind. *Matter* refers to the outside world and sensory knowledge where

the *mind* has to with consciousness
and thoughts.

- External perception opposed to
internal perception. External
perception is the one arising from the
interaction of five senses and worldly
objects, while internal perception is
described as the one comes of inner
sense mainly the mind.

- Observation as a mean to reach
conclusions which are only true if
they can be justified with reason.

- With the limited time and energy
humans have, they only learn a
fraction of facts, truths and
knowledge of this world, unless they
cooperate with each other to rapidly

acquire and share knowledge and to enrich each other's lives.

- Human soul is formed from three main elements each element is called "Guna". The concept says that human have different proportions of the three gunas (goodness – passion – darkness) and that the fundamental nature and psychological dispositions of beings is a consequence of the relative proportion of these three gunas.

When goodness predominates an individual, the qualities of wisdom, constructiveness, and peacefulness manifest; when passion predominates, craving, passion-driven activity and restlessness manifest; and when darkness predominates, ignorance, delusion, destruction and suffering manifest. This yoga concept is about balance and dominance of best element of the soul.

- A philosophical concept suggests that guna of "Goodness" comes from consciousness or *mind,* while "darkness" comes from *matter* or the physical world.

Chapter 1: Why Practice Yoga? The Benefits & Types

After a brief introduction on the broad term, the discipline and the philosophy "Yoga", in this chapter we will go through benefits, usages and types of yoga. By the end of this chapter you will be able to set your objectives for practicing yoga and consequently, choosing the type which helps you best get your aim fulfilled.

1. Benefits

The benefits of yoga are numerous, so we will categorize them within three major aspects; health, physical abilities, psychological wellness and self-development.

1.1 Health:

- *Increases blood flow:*

Yoga helps with blood flow, circulation, levels of hemoglobin and red blood cells and the reach of oxygen to body cells.

Later on in this book we will discuss poses; twisting poses wring out venous blood from internal organs and allow oxygenated blood to flow. Inverted poses, such as Headstand, Handstand, and Shoulder-stand, encourage venous blood from the legs and pelvis to flow back to the heart, and in the lungs it gets freshly oxygenated.

It helps with swelling in legs from heart or kidney problems. Furthermore, it decreases risks of heart attacks and strokes, as it thins the blood by making platelets less sticky and by cutting the level of clot-promoting proteins in the blood.

- Strengthens lymphatic system and boosts immunity:

Yoga, through stretching muscles and moving organs, helps the lymphatic system fight infection, destroy cancerous cells, and dispose of the toxic waste products of cellular functioning.

- Drops high blood pressure:

All yoga positions that have to do with relaxation and lying down help drop high blood pressure.

- Lowers cortisol levels:

High cortisol levels compromise the immune system, undermine memory, cause depression, increase blood pressure, result in "food-seeking behavior" and consequently result in weight gain, risk of diabetes and heart attack.

1.2 Physical abilities:

- Flexibility:

Obviously, yoga takes your body to a whole new level of flexibility. After few weeks you reach your toes and even do a backbend. Yoga gets you a more flexible spine, knee joints and thighs.

- *Strong muscles:*

Yoga builds muscles without affecting flexibility. They improve muscles abilities which can help you on the long term with aging.

- *Right posture:*

Driving, setting in front of computers all day and even sleeping in a wrong way can affect your posture, hurt your nick and back and get you a constant feel of pain and tiredness. Yoga helps with correct posture, balanced head weight, correct nick angle and erected spine.

- Better bone density:

Many yoga positions require carrying the whole body using certain parts, like arms or shoulders. This helps bones density.

- Improved balance:

People with bad posture or dysfunctional movement patterns usually have poor proprioception (the ability to feel what your body is doing and where it is going). Yoga improve proprioception and thus balance.

-Eases back pain:

Working on stiffed muscles and wrong postures mean less back pain.

1.3 Psychology:

- Stress relief:

Yoga and meditation help with stress relief where people can take a break of the fast-pace world and sit or lay down relaxing and meditating.

- Inner Peace:

Meditation is all about finding peace and a quite spot inside your own soul to go to and just mute your mind and loud fears and to enjoy a relaxed self.

- Mental health:

Less stress and inner peace is basically immunity against depression, low energy and lack of interest and passion.

- Focus:

Being less distracted with your thoughts means more concentrated, problem solver, quick thinker and a person with strong memory and high IQ.

- Better sleep:

Less stress and less tiredness mean deep and good sleep.

1.4 Self-development:

- Healthy life style:

Yoga helps for a healthier life style as it makes you move and have inner strength to give up bad eating habits.

- Higher self-esteem:

Yoga helps people get rid of their negative and stressing ideas, it also helps them look within their souls and see their worth and value.

- Inner strength and motivation:

Yoga helps in find the strength and motivation to change. Giving bad habits and taking new life style.

- Better relationships:

A person who is good terms with their own self and have less stress and more peace can build a healthier relationship and better communication.

- Self-care and awareness:

Practicing yoga regularly gets you in the mood of that only you is caring for this self and that body. It helps you to be aware of your health and to make the necessary changes in your life.

2. Usages:

So after you read many benefits for yoga, you will need to focus on the usages that meet your own needs and objectives. Are you practicing for weight loss, better body shape and strength, stress relief, healing (back/shoulder/nick/knee pain) or for self-improvement and inner peace? You can still have more than one usage in mind while we next discuss yoga types and help us find you your best fit.

3. Types of yoga:

Anusara

Anusara is a kind of a new type of yoga. It was first introduced in 1997 by John Friend. It is about the "celebration of heart", and it is based on opening our heart and maximize the goodness guna through slightly difficult poses like back bend. It usually has a teacher to lead student into inner self.

Ashtanga

Ashtanga was introduced to the West in 1970. It is a physically demanding style where certain poses are practices every time in the exact same order. This is a hot and sweaty discipline. It is also called power yoga.

Bikram

Bikram Yoga was founded by gold medal Olympic weight lifter Bikram Choudhury in 1963. Which doesn't make so surprising to know that this discipline is very tough and physical demanding. Same poses in same sequences are practiced in 95-105 degree temperature. Bikram yoga maximizes muscular strength, muscular endurance, cardiovascular flexibility and weight loss which makes a very popular discipline.

Hatha

Hatha yoga can be used to refer to any discipline of yoga that basically includes slow and simple poses, meditation and self-realization. It is very popular in the United Sates and really suitable for beginners and for those who want a mix of physical postures and stress relief.

Lyengar

Lyngar yoga was developed by yoga master, B.K.S. Lyengar, more than 60 years ago. It is about finding the right alignment promoting strength, flexibility, endurance, and balance through coordinated breathing and poses that require precise body alignment. The poses are generally held longer than in other styles of yoga before stretching into another. Equipment like cushions, blankets, straps, and blocks are used. Everyone - even the elderly, sick, and disabled - can practice it, because of its slow pace, attention to detail, and use of props. Iyengar yoga can be especially good if you're recovering from an injury and one of the most popular types of yoga taught today.

Restorative

Restorative yoga is basically to relax in a beneficial pose for your body. Restorative classes use bolsters, blankets, and blocks where people just relax their body and mind.

Vinyasa

One of the most common yoga styles. Vinyasa means "flow", and it is a flow of intensive practices, movements and poses. Music is usually played to keep things lively. The intensity of the Vinyasa is similar to Ashtanga, but vinyasa classes are diverse.

Kundalini

Kundalini concentrates on awakening the energy at the base of the spine and drawing it upward. It is pretty intense. In addition to postures there are also chanting, meditation, and breathing exercises.

Viniyoga

Viniyoga is commonly used for therapeutic purposes. In cases of injuries or of recovering from a surgery. It is a gentle, healing practice that is tailored to each person's body type and needs as they grow and change.

After reading about different styles and setting your objectives you can now pick the perfect style for you. If you want fitness and to get in shape as well as to explore the mind-body connection Ashtanga yoga, or Bikram yoga.

If you have an injury, a medical condition, or other limitations, start with a slower class that focuses on alignment, such as Iyengar yoga or viniyoga.

If meditation and spirituality are your primary goal, then try one of the yoga styles that include plenty of meditation, chanting, and the philosophic aspects such as kundalini yoga.

And finally you have those types who mixes more than one approach to maximize benefits.

Chapter 2: How to start? "Guidelines"

In this chapter we are moving to guidelines and preparations, so you get everything ready before getting down to business.

1. Choosing the time:

It is not important what time to practice but rather how frequent and how long. It means you don't have to choose daytime or evening but instead duration and frequency. Consistency is so important. You can practice for short duration but daily that's better than irregular longer practice.

Everyday practice will help build concentration, increase flexibility and strengthen willpower, making it easier to practice the next day.

The duration is minimum of 10 minutes, however; 15-25 is the ideal regular short practice to cover variety of poses and get deep in meditation. It is necessary to have a couple of longer session each week.

The exact time can be fixed every day or changing. The most important thing is to find a time with clear mind, not being rushed or in a hurry. You should also see what time suits your body better, is it in the morning or in in the evening. Some might find their muscles tight in the morning, and others find workout difficult before sleeping time.

So find your own time of the day, practice regularly at least 10 minutes and preferably 25 minutes. If you think you can go to a regular class that can help.

2. Choosing the place:

Find yourself a clear spot so you stretch freely in all the directions. The place needs to be comfortably heated and well ventilated. Another important aspect when choosing the place is quietness. Make sure there is no possible interruption or noise. Switch off or make silent all the devices, and make sure kids or pets are playing away from your spot.

3. Choosing clothes:

Make sure to wear comfortable, warm and kind of fit cloth. Shorts are preferred. Wear a sport bra and a tight shirt, so it doesn't slide to your head during certain poses. Clothing such as: leotards, cotton tights, bike shorts, loose T-shirts or tank tops would be good.

Tie your hair so it doesn't bother you during poses or got you hot.

Yoga is practiced bare-foot.

4. Choosing equipment:

Mats:

The mat helps you define your personal space, creates traction for your hands and feet so you don't slip and also provides a bit of cushioning on a hard floor. In order to choose the right mat think what you want; to feel the floor, to have a thick thing between you and the floor or a portable to carry with you.

A standard yoga mat is about 1/8 inch thick, while the thick ones are 1/4 inch. There are also "travel yoga mats," that are a mere 1/16 inch thick. They fold easily and don't weigh much, which is a best choice for people who care about mobility.

Blankets:

Use folded blankets for both warmth and padding for a variety of yoga postures. The can be used to sit or lie on.

Blocks:

Blocks will be helpful at the beginning when you still can't reach for the floor by yourself. They sport your hands or legs. They also provide support for limbs or even the back to improve flexibility and alignment.

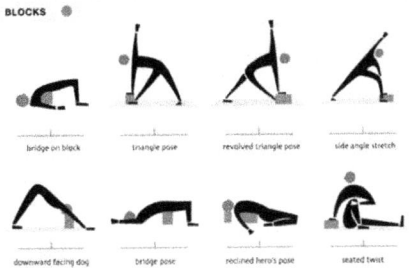

BLOCKS

| bridge on block | triangle pose | revolved triangle pose | side angle stretch |

| downward facing dog | bridge pose | reclined hero's pose | seated twist |

Straps:

Straps help you reach for your feet or hands and get your body parts connected when your flexibility is not enough. They help in keeping right postures and stretching body limbs.

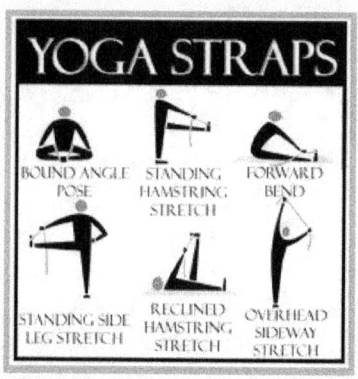

Now we have everything done let's
start!

Chapter 3: Breathing

Starting from this chapter the real journey begins. We will help you with the real practice. First we will discuss breathing in this chapter then we will move to meditation, warm ups and finally postures. By the end of this chapter you will be able to start the first step and one of the most important in practicing yoga both the physical and spiritual sides.

First thing in starting yoga or "asana" is to take a breath. Breathing might sound an obvious part that doesn't need explanations – I mean we all breathe! –

However, most people are only "chest breathers" expanding only the upper chest when they inhale and that means they use only a fraction of their full breathing capacity. People can turn into chest breathers as a result of a combination of stress, poor posture, long hours behind desks, and flat-stomach phobia. Chest breathing causes imbalance in the oxygen/carbon dioxide ratio, which results in hyperventilation and dizziness.

In order to breathe correctly, breath needs to be rhythmic, slow and complete. Use the diaphragm and ribs to fill and empty the lungs. With a proper movement of the diaphragm your breath will be correct.

Importance

Once again, let go of the obvious reference for breathing. Of course you need to breathe to stay alive. However, proper breathing can give you great benefits. Deep abdominal breathing allows a full exchange of air, keeping the oxygen/carbon dioxide ratio balanced, tone up your entire system and enhance health and vitality.

Giving great attention to every part of breathing process is important to maximize benefits. Inhalation and exhalation establish a constant flow and release of energy within us. While inhalation provide your body with energy, exhalation relaxes it.

Breathing in yoga

In yoga, breathing element is known as prana or life-force. Prana does not just refer to the oxygen itself, but rather to the subtle life-giving element extracted from the breathing process. *"The more life-force you have in your body, the more "alive" you are; the less life-force, the less "life"."* That is how yoga coaches emphasize on the importance of Prana element.

Breathing is a vital element in achieving the objectives of yoga both physically and spiritually. Practicing yoga breathing, or breath control is called pranayama in yogic terms. The word "Pranayama" can be broken into two parts: Prana means life force and Yama means control. Yoga have certain techniques to reach a conscious control of the breath and to create a proper rhythm of slow, deep breathing.

Yoga depends on Pranayama breathing exercises as the link between the physical and the mental disciplines of yoga. Because the breath, body and mind are so closely linked, and a change in one of them immediately affects the other two.

Furthermore, yogic breathing exercises help to keep the two sides of the brain in balance, so it is not just a link between the body and soul but also between the different sides of our brain. Each half of the brain deals with different functions and different aspects.

The right side of the brain is calming, intuitive, inner-directed and emotional, which deals with simultaneous reasoning and spatial and nonverbal activities. While the left side of the brain is aggressive, logical, outer-directed, rational and objective which deals with sequential reasoning and mathematical and verbal activities. Proper breathing helps the two sides of the brain to work together.

Another things is that proper breathing soothes the nervous system, improves concentration and increases the ability to deal with complex situations without stress. It also increases emotional stability, combats depression and helps in the relief of grief and sadness.

So basically controlling breath can lead to controlling energy within the body, and ultimately to full control over the mind.

"Yogic breathing energizes and cleanses the body, calms and relaxes the mind, and serves as a perfect warm-up for practicing yoga poses. In coordination with yoga poses, the breath unifies mind and body, balances opposing energies, and helps the body relax deeply and safely into each pose."

Breathing techniques:

In all your breathing exercises you can sit comfortably in a cross-legged position or lie flat on your back. When sitting, you can use any of the previous mentioned equipment for support; a folded blanket or a cushion under the buttocks would do. Hands can be relaxed by your sides, on your legs or can be placed on the abdomen to feel the rising and falling during the flow of air. Remember always to relax your mind and body.

Abdominal Breathing

Inhale slowly and deeply through the nose. Feel the abdomen expand while the chest is still. Exhale slowly. Feel the abdomen sink down. Repeat the process ten times (one inhalation and one exhalation count as only one breath.)

Benefit: it brings air to the lowest part of the lungs, exercises the diaphragm and enhance breathing capacity. It also massages internal organs and it helps with stress and calming emotions, and as a result induces restful sleep.

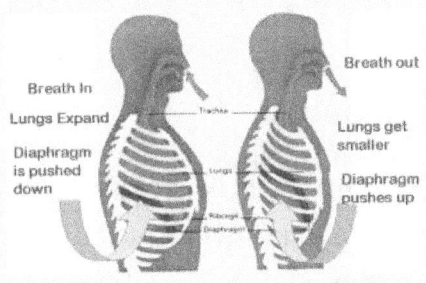

Rib Cage Breathing

Gently contract the abdomen. Inhale slowly through the nose into the rib cage. Do not pull the breath deep into your lungs; instead, keep it focused between your ribs. Feel the ribs expand outward, as you inhale, and inward, as you exhale. Repeat five times.

Benefit: Relaxes the mind and body and strengthens the lungs.

Complete Breathing

Inhale slowly through the nose, feel the abdomen expand first, then the rib cage, and finally feel the air filling the upper chest. Slowly exhale, emptying the lungs from top to bottom. Your shoulders and head should stay essentially in the same position throughout. Do not hold your breath either at the top or the bottom of the breath but make the transition smooth. Inhalation is done from the bottom up and exhalation from the top down. Repeat five times.

Benefit: combats tensions and stress. It can be used anywhere, anytime to calm your mind and help quiet physical responses to stress - rapid heartbeat and breathing, and tense muscles. Use this technique to center yourself before your meditation and before asana practice to make them even more effective.

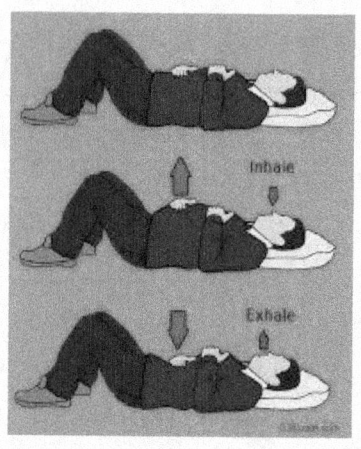

Alternate Nostril Breathing

Extend the thumb, ring finger and little finger of your right hand and fold down your other fingers. Close your right nostril with your thumb and inhale slowly and deeply through the left nostril for a count of 8. Then press the ring and pinky fingers against the left side of the nose, sealing the left nostril closed while keeping the thumb against the right nostril, and hold for a count of 8.

Lift the thumb from the right side of the nose, opening the right nostril. Exhale slowly and fully through the right nostril for a count of 8. Inhale slowly and deeply through the right nostril, still holding the left nostril shut for a count of 8. Cover the right nostril with the thumb and hold for a count of 8. Release the left nostril and exhale through the left nostril for a count of 8. Repeat sequence five times.

Benefit: helps with balance between the mind and body, relaxation and concentration.

Alternate Nostril Breathing

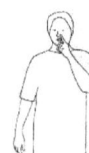 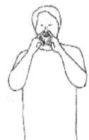 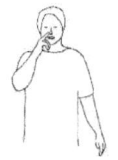 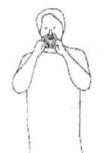

Close left nostril by placing left forefinger on that nostril and breathing in through right nostril.	Close right nostril, so that both nostrils are closed simultaneously.	Release only left finger and breathe out through left nostril, then breathe in through same nostril.	Close left nostril and then releases right nostril and repeat the same exercise 3 times.

Extract from YOU & ME Breathing Techniques for Special Needs, p35. Maria Gunstone, 2005

Ujjayi Breath

Inhale slowly, keeping the mouth closed. Partially close or contract the back of your throat to slow down the breath. Hold for a few seconds. Exhale, again partially closing or contracting at the back of the throat. This breath will make a hoarse hiss-like sound like steam being released from a radiator. Repeat five times.

Benefit: Increases lung capacity, opens the chest, relaxes the nervous system, increases oxygen in the blood, reduces phlegm and strengthens the immune system.

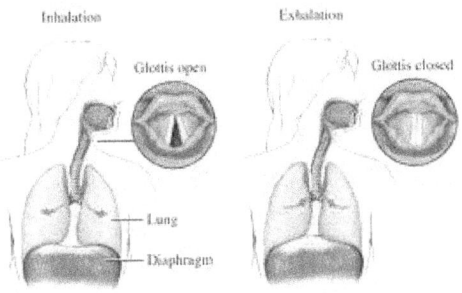

Chapter 4: Meditation

Moving to the main part focusing on mind and soul. Meditation will get you relaxed and enhance your mind concentrations abilities.

First, you need to know that meditation and yoga are not the same thing or integrated. You can do yoga without meditation or do meditation without yoga. However, they both compatible and lead to one another. To maximize yoga benefits do some meditations before it for 5 to 10 minutes. Moreover, yoga helps with concentration and with peace of mind, so basically it leads to better meditation and great results out of it.

People might confuse meditation with deep silence and quietness of the mind. Basically, meditation is not a deep sleep or total shut down, but more an active mind with great efforts taken to achieve certain status of concentration.

Meditation is all about focusing on the present. It starts with focus on a certain object then develops into the cessation of all other thought and it ends with quietness of mind and peace.

While the techniques and the steps are not that difficult, meditation requires patience, understanding and practice. Keeping the mind focus and going deep through the present moment is the hard part.

Try not to expect any particular result. High expectations always come with disappointments. Do not give up quickly. Even if you think nothing is happening and you find it boring to sit still, consistency and the daily effort will get you comfortable with the status and will increase concentration and you will be able to gain control over your mind.

Control of the mind is something worth effort and patience. It is a key to success in life. Meditation will also help you with find a peaceful spot within you to combat stress, depression and difficult moments. A clear mind will get you more active in any activity you do and help you with decision making.

Meditations techniques:

With all your meditation techniques get in seated pose. Do some breathing and of course keep in mind all the previous mentioned instructions about time, place, duration and consistency. Since meditation is about concentration, the techniques will only differ with the object to concentrate on.

Mantra meditation

This technique focuses on sound. This sound can be any sound, but it also can be phrases prayers of affirmations. It can be both silently from your side with a teacher or a recording, or it can be you the one who think of our say loudly the phrase, prayer or affirmation. Find words or prayers that calm you, and when you go to the class make sure the teacher knows you well. Once you have chosen a mantra, do not change it.

Examples: "Om", "peace", "love", or "joy"; "I am relaxed" or "I am calm and alert" Think "I am" as you breathe in and "relaxed" as you breathe out.

Imagery or Visualization

Visualize an object that relaxes you such as a flower, the ocean, a clear sky or any object. Keep your eyes closed and visualize that image until you feel relaxed. After that, slowly let go of the image but keep the quiet as long as you can. Go back to your image whenever you need, but be careful so you don't get so involved in the image and any memories or perceptions associated it.

Breath Counting Meditation

Use the breath as the point of focus. Observe every nuance of the breath and each sensation it produces: how it moves in your abdomen and torso, how it feels as it moves, its quality, its temperature, and so on. Or you may mentally think "in" inhaling and "out" exhaling. Another way to observe the breath is to count it. Breathe in for 3 to 7 counts and breathe out for the same length of time. You can use earplugs to increase your concentration on the sound of your breath.

Chapter 5: Warm-ups and postures

By this point you might feel FINALLY! I will do real yoga here. Remember that postures are just the physical part of yoga and to be really effective should be combined with breathing and meditation or it will just be a kind of a work-out. We will start discussing poses and we will start with simple ones as warm-ups retrieved from: www.yogabasics.com.

Warm-up 1:

1. Start in Easy Pose or Accomplished Pose.

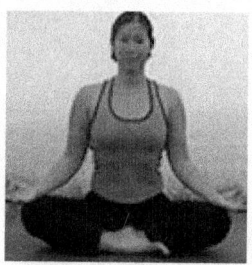

Keep the shoulders down and back, the spine long and the chest open.

2. Inhale the fingertips up to the ceiling.

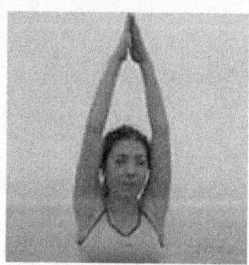

Keep the shoulders down and back, the hips grounded to the floor and reach through the fingertips.

3. Exhale and round forward with the palms to the floor.

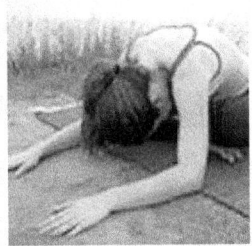

Round the spine and relax the head and elbows down.

4. Inhale the fingertips up to the ceiling.

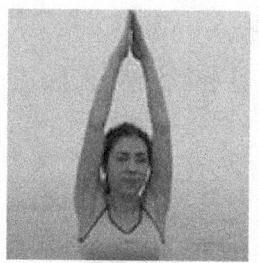

Keep the shoulders down and back, the hips grounded to the floor and reach through the fingertips.

5. Exhale and twist to the left.

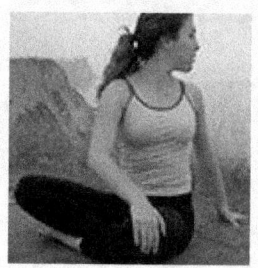

Place the left hand on the right knee and the right hand behind your back. Look over your right shoulder and look behind you. Keep the spine long and the shoulders down.

6. Inhale the fingertips up to the ceiling.

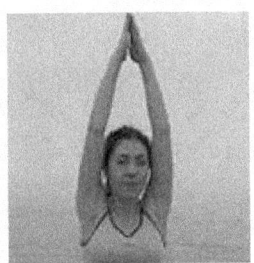

Keep the shoulders down and back, the hips grounded to the floor and reach through the fingertips.

7. Exhale and twist to the right.

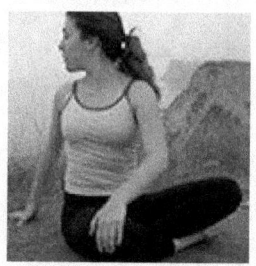

Place the right hand on the left knee and the left hand behind your back. Look over your left shoulder and look behind you. Keep the spine long and the shoulders down.

8. Inhale the fingertips up to the ceiling.

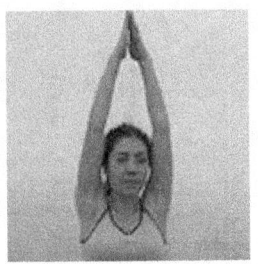

Keep the shoulders down and back,
the hips grounded to the floor and
reach through the fingertips.

9. Exhale the left hand to the floor
and arch to the left.

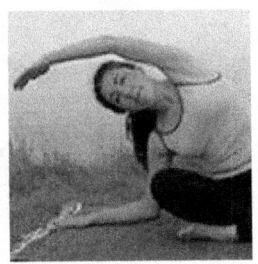

Reach out through the right fingers and lower the left elbow as close to the floor as comfortable. Keep the chin off the chest and the right arm over the right ear.

10. Inhale the fingertips up to the ceiling.

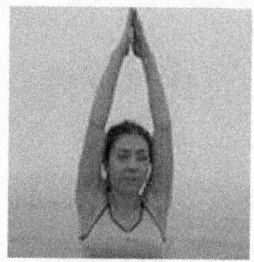

Keep the shoulders down and back, the hips grounded to the floor and reach through the fingertips.

11. Exhale the right hand to the floor and arch to the right.

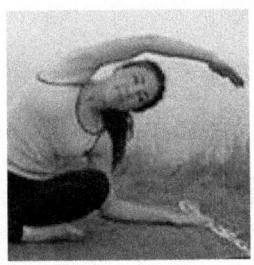

Reach out through the left fingers and lower the right elbow as close to the floor as comfortable. Keep the chin off the chest and the right arm over the left ear.

12. Inhale the fingertips up to the ceiling.

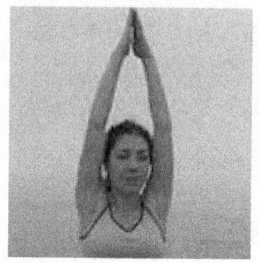

Keep the shoulders down and back, the hips grounded to the floor and reach through the fingertips.

13. Exhale the hands forward and round the spine.

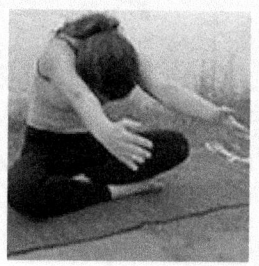

Reach out through the fingertips, drop the head down and round the spine.

14. Inhale the arms behind you.

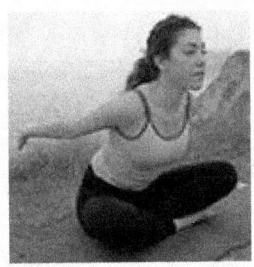

Reach back through the fingertips to draw the shoulder blades together. Press forward through the chest and look up towards the ceiling.

15. Exhale the hands to the knees or floor.

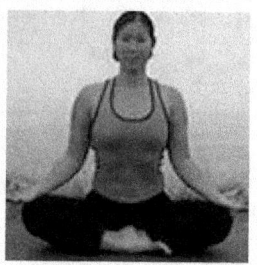

Bring the spine back to neutral position. Keep the shoulders down and back, the spine long and the chest open.

Warm-up 2:

1. Start in Easy Pose

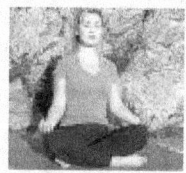

A. Inhale and press the hips down and reach the crown up to lengthen the spine. Roll the shoulders down and back to open the chest. Relax the face and rest the tongue on the roof of the mouth.

B. Lengthen the inhalation and exhalation by breathing deeply into the belly through the nose. Release any thoughts or distractions and let the mind be focused on the breath.

C. Breathe and hold for 10-30 breaths.

2. Come into Table position on your hands and knees

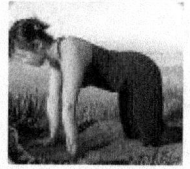

A. Place the palms under the shoulders and the knees under the hips.

B. The back is flat and the gaze is between the hands.

C. Press back through the tailbone and forward through the crown of the head to lengthen the spine.

3. Inhale into Dog Tilt

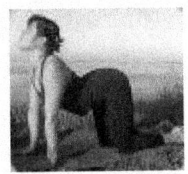

A. Reach the tailbone up towards the ceiling by arching the spine and letting the belly drop towards the floor.

B. Press down into the palms to drop the shoulders away from the ears and look up at the ceiling.

4. Exhale into Cat Tilt

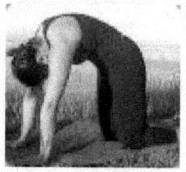

A. Tuck the tailbone under by rounding the spine and pulling the belly up towards the spine.

B. Press down into the palms to reach the middle of the back up towards the ceiling. Let the head hang from the neck.

5. Repeat #3 and #4 moving with the breath 3-6 times

6. From Dog tilt, exhale into Downward Facing Dog

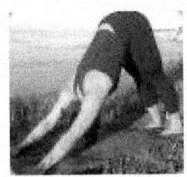

A. Tuck the toes under, bend the elbows and lift the hips up and back.

B. Press firmly into the hands and arms to press the hips back. Let the head hang from the neck.

C. Press the heels into the floor. The legs are straight or can be slightly bent to flatten the back.

D. Breathe and hold for 3-6 breaths.

7. Inhale and step right forward into Low Warrior

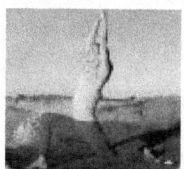

A. Step the foot between the two hands with the knee directly over the ankle. Lower the back knee and top of foot to the floor.

B. Press down into the palms, fingertips or fists to lift the crown up and to lengthen the spine. Roll the shoulders down and back and press the chest forward. Press the front knee forward and let the hips sink towards the floor, lightly stretching the insides of the legs.

C. Press the legs down into the floor as you lift out of the waist reaching the crown and fingertips up towards the ceiling.

D. Breathe and hold for 2-5 breaths.

8. Exhale the palms to the floor and step back into Downward Facing Dog

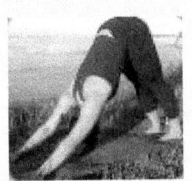

A. Tuck the toes under, bend the elbows and lift the hips up and back.

B. Press firmly into the hands and arms to press the hips back. Let the head hang from the neck.

C. Press the heels into the floor. The legs are straight or can be slightly bent to flatten the back.

D. Breathe and hold for 3-6 breaths.

9. Step left foot forward, repeating #7 through #9 on opposite side

10. Exhale and bend the knees to the floor into Child Pose

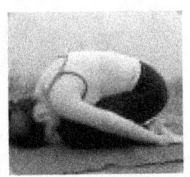

A. Press the hips to the heels with the tops of the feet flat to the floor. Let the forehead rest on the floor and allow the body to completely relax.

B. Breathe deeply into the belly for 3-6 breaths.

11. Slide the arms forward and scoop into Cobra

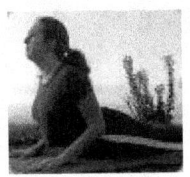

A. Press the palms flat to the floor directly under the shoulders to lift the crown up. Relax the shoulders down and back to press the chest forward.

B. If the back feels strained, bend the elbows more or come onto the forearms.

C. Breathe and hold for 2-5 breath

12. Exhale and lower the chest to the floor, inhale lift into Half Locust

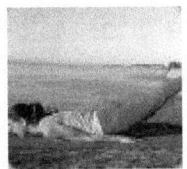

A. Slide the arms alongside the body with the palms down. If comfortable, rock from side to side to bring the arms under the torso.

B. With the chin on the floor, inhale and press the arms and hips down into the floor and lengthen the legs by reaching out through the toes. Engaging the core and lower body, lift the legs up as high as comfortable without strain.

C. Breathe and hold for 2-5 breaths.

13. Exhale and lower to the floor, roll over on your back into Shavasana

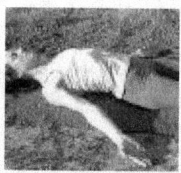

A. Let the arms and legs flop out to the sides. The arms are 6-8 inches from the sides of your body and the palms are facing up.

B. Close the eyes and consciously relax the body from the toes to the crown of the head.

C. Breathe deeply through the nose into the belly, and stay in the pose for 10-15 minutes.

14. End in Easy Pose

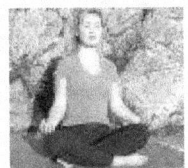

2. Poses:

Standing Postures

Standing poses provide strength and mobility to the hips, knees, neck, and shoulders. On a psychological level, standing poses create confidence, enhance willpower, and strengthen character.

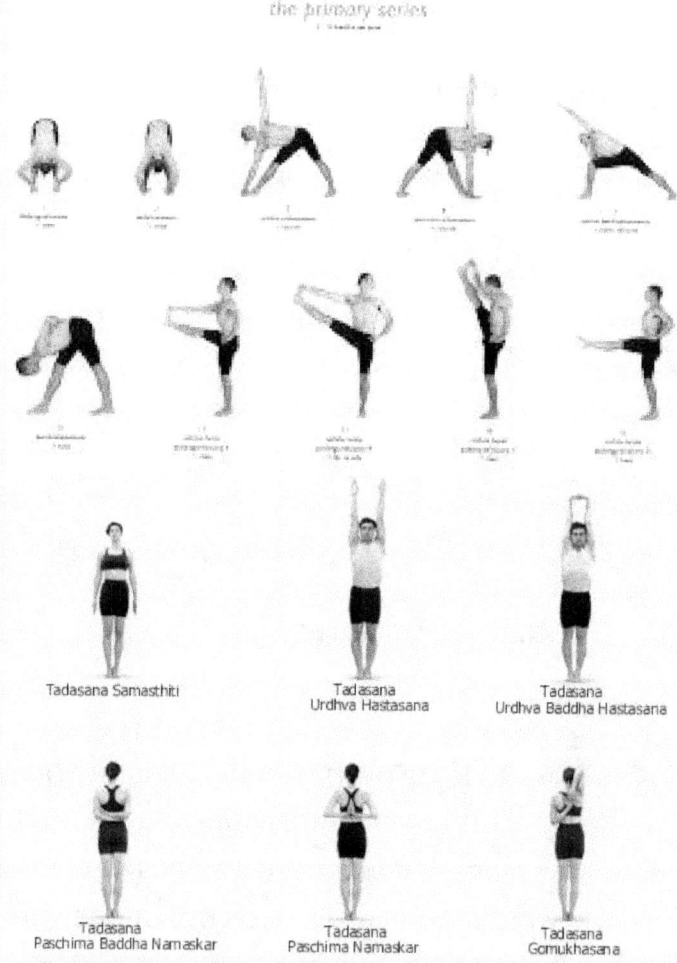

the primary series

Tadasana Samasthiti

Tadasana
Urdhva Hastasana

Tadasana
Urdhva Baddha Hastasana

Tadasana
Paschima Baddha Namaskar

Tadasana
Paschima Namaskar

Tadasana
Gomukhasana

Seated Postures

Seated poses are beneficial in increasing flexibility in the lower back, hips and hamstrings. They also calming.

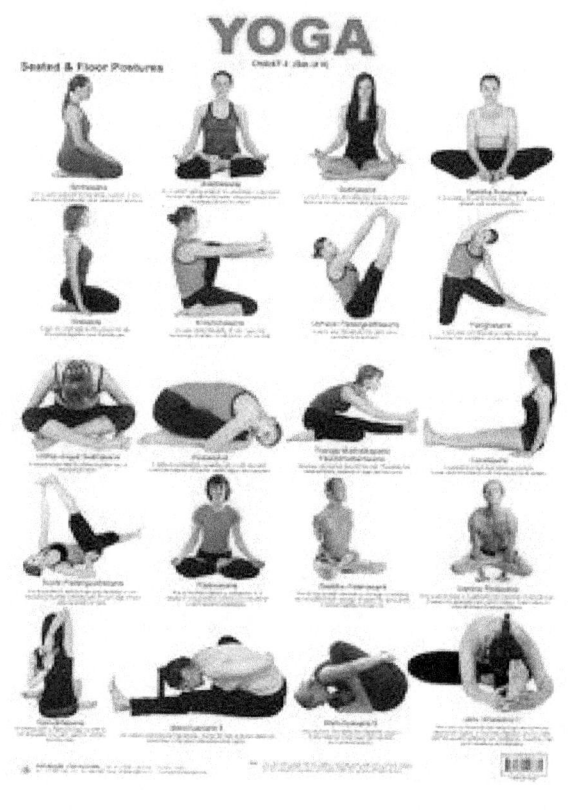

84

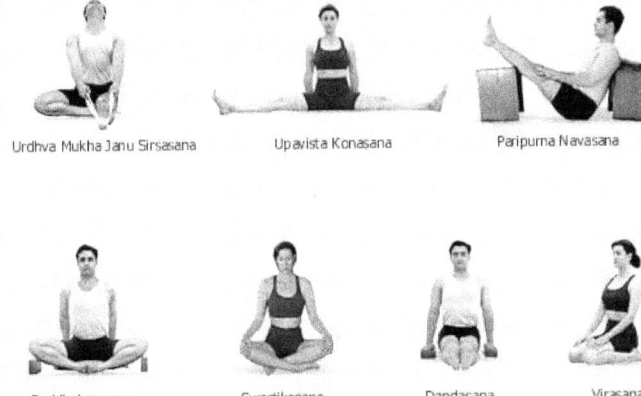

Urdhva Mukha Janu Sirsasana   Upavista Konasana   Paripurna Navasana

Baddhakonasana   Swastikasana   Dandasana   Virasana

Reclining Postures

Reclining postures are two
categories: prone and supine poses.
The prone poses are done facing the
floor, either on the hands and knees
or lying on the stomach, while Supine
poses are done while lying on the

back. These poses are relaxing and restful. Reclining poses help to stretch the abdomen and increase the mobility of the spine and hips.

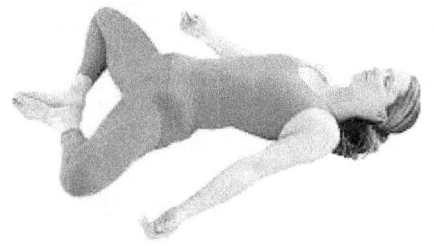

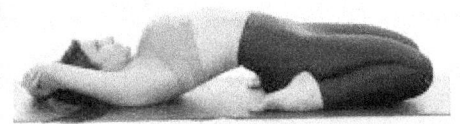

Forward and back Bends

Forward bends improve the blood circulation, aid digestion and calm the emotions. They stretch the lower back and lengthen the hamstrings, while backbends strengthen the arms and shoulders and increase flexibility of the spine.

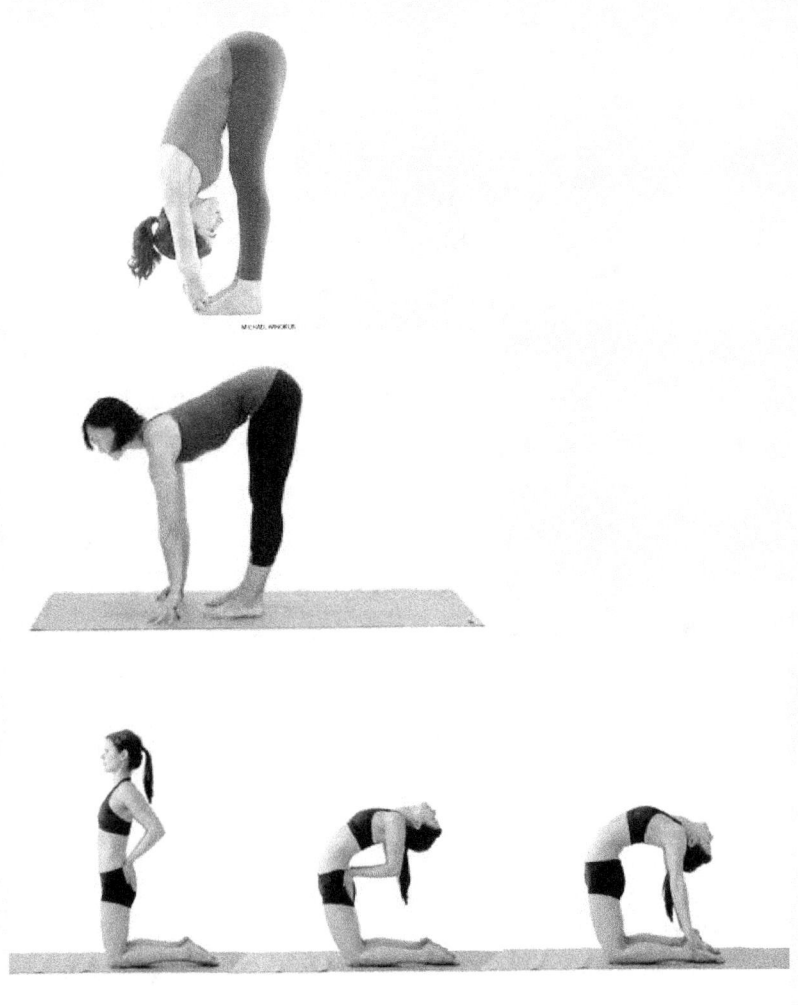

Twists

Twists increase the flexibility of the spine, hips and upper back. This group of postures also tones and stimulates the abdominal organs aiding digestion and relieving constipation. Twisting postures are advised to be done after a series of sitting poses or forward bends, which gives the hips and spine a proper warm-up. When done after backbends, they tend to relieve any lower back discomfort.

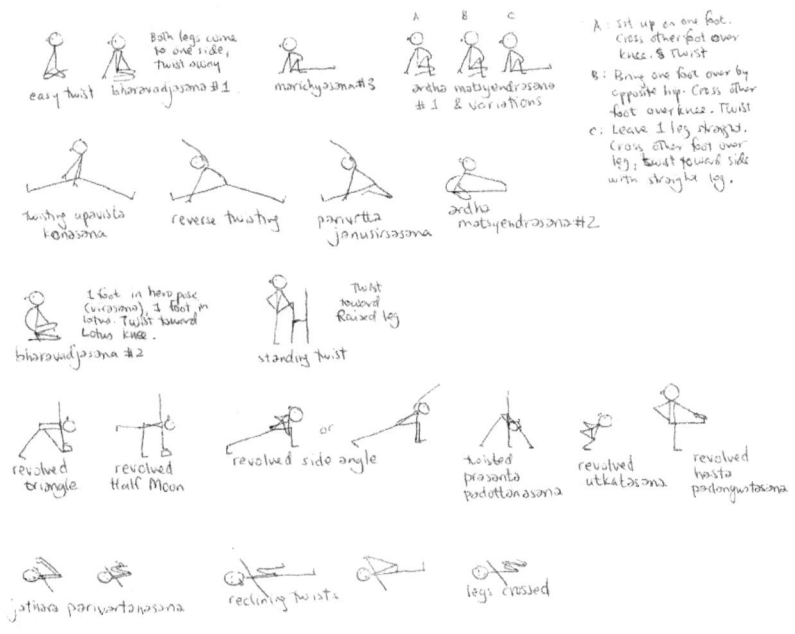

TWISTING POSES

easy twist — bharavadjasana #1 — Both legs come to one side, Twist away — marichyasana #3 — ardha matsyendrasana #1 & variations

A: Sit up on one foot. Cross other foot over knee. & Twist
B: Bring one foot over by opposite hip. Cross other foot over knee. Twist
C: Leave 1 leg straight. Cross other foot over leg; twist toward side with straight leg.

twisting upavista konasana — reverse twisting — parivrtta janusirsasana — ardha matsyendrasana #2

bharavadjasana #2 — 1 foot in hero pose (virasana), 1 foot in lotus. Twist toward Lotus knee. — standing twist — Twist toward Raised leg

revolved triangle — revolved Half Moon — revolved side angle or — twisted prasarita padottanasana — revolved utkatasana — revolved hasta padangustasana

jathara parivartanasana — reclining twists — legs crossed

Inverted Postures

Inverted postures reverse gravity, bringing fresh blood to the head and heart, thus revitalizing the mind and the whole body. These poses tone

91

the internal organs and glandular system, stimulate brain function, improve circulation and refresh tired legs.

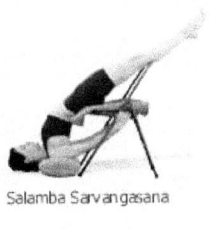

Salamba Sarvangasana

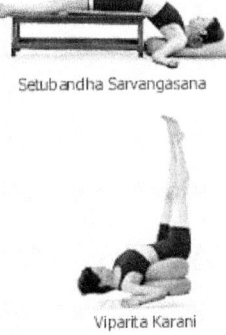

Setubandha Sarvangasana

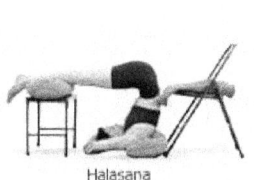

Halasana

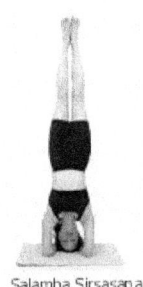

Salamba Sirsasana

Viparita Karani

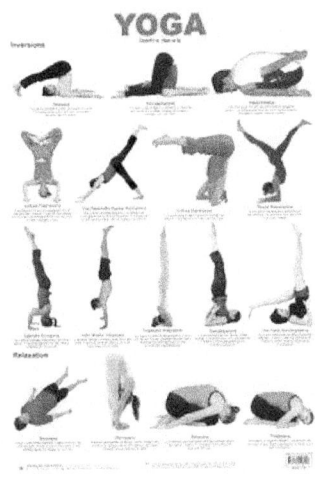

Balancing Postures

Balancing postures help with lightness, strength and agility. They also help develop body control, muscle tone, coordination, and concentration.

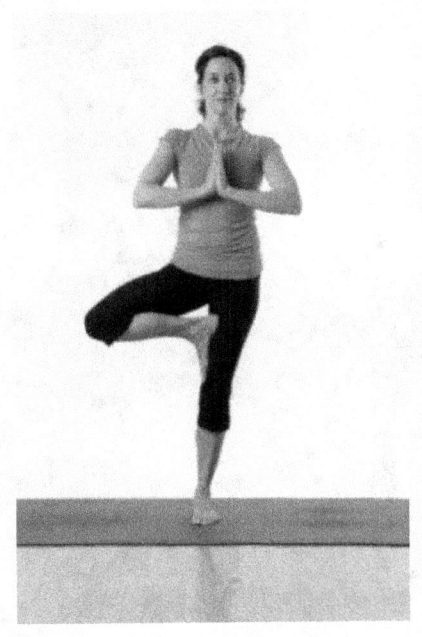

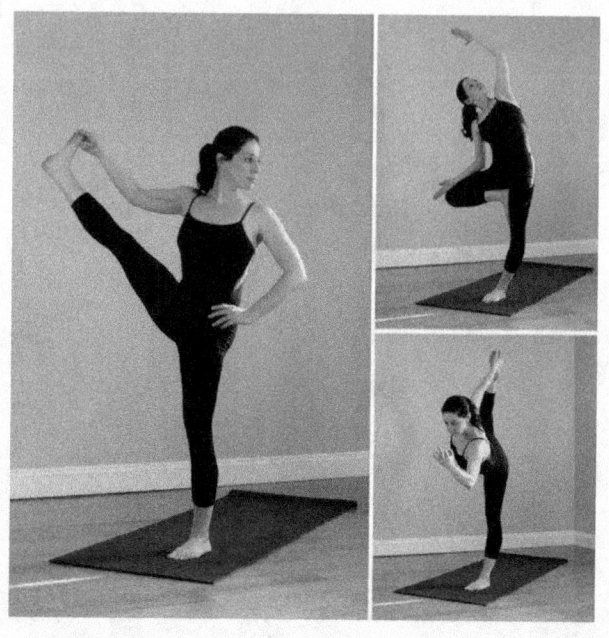

3. Application

Make sure when choosing the kind of sequence to recognize your body's capabilities and limits. Ease yourself gently into each position, and when you are holding a pose, check the body to see if you can feel tension building up anywhere. If you do, consciously try to relax that tension using the breath.

Always begin with 2 - 3 warm-up postures, such as Mountain, Downward Facing Dog or Sun Salutation, as they stretch the spine, arms and legs. Then you can move on to more strenuous poses that strengthen the body and increase endurance. Standing, inverted and backbend poses would apply here.

Your session should include some poses from all the major groupings; standing, inversions, twists, forward bends, and backbends.

While in the pose, do not hold the breath. Between postures, take 1 to 2 breaths to quiet the mind.

Moving from one pose to another without breaking form is called "sequencing". This method of practice allows for a balanced workout regardless of practice length. Sequences can consist of related poses for the purpose of energizing (as with standing poses or backbends) or relaxing (with forward bends or restorative poses) the body or working on specific areas such as the hips, shoulders, or feet.

At the end of your practice it is important to take 5 to 10 minutes to relax your body. Relaxation is a state of total receptivity where, through deep breathing, the body can replenish and rejuvenate itself as the natural potential of the body to heal itself comes into play. Always end with several minutes in Corpse Pose to renew both mind and body.

Your sequence can be adjusted to your practice to your schedule and feelings. Some days you may not feel as energetic or flexible or you may feel weak or tired. On those days, try doing restorative poses, such as supine poses and forward bends.

Always remember that consistency is the key to success. Be patient with yourself and don't rush to find results. *"Yoga can be a life-long pursuit, but persistency, consistency and discipline are required to gain the many lasting benefits yoga offers."*

www.ingramcontent.com/pod-product-compliance
Lightning Source LLC
Chambersburg PA
CBHW062042280526
45788CB00003B/1086